THE UNIQUE AND PERFECT GUIDE ON IRRITABLE BOWEL SYNDROME (IBS)

Detailed guide on how to Purchase THE UNIQUE AND PERFECT GUIDE ON IRRITABLE BOWEL SYNDROME(IBS) Legally & Cheap; Without Doctor's Prescription

By:

DOCTOR ELIZA PARKER

Copyright@2018

TABLE OF CONTENTS

CHAPTER ONE

DETAINS ABOUT IBS

The term irritable bowel syndrome, which is abbreviated as IBS,or spastic colon, is one of a gastrointestinal disorder in a human body which affect both adult and children. Persons with IBS experiences Abdominal Pain, Cramping, Intolerance to Food etc.

IBS is simply when your digestive system has some disordering.

The main attribute or causes of IBS is not known and many factors may be responsible to its cause. This disease comes in different form which are:

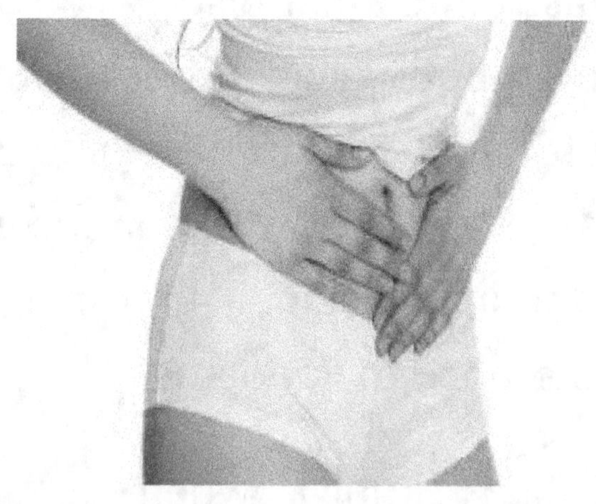

❖ IBS accompanied with Diarrhea(IBS-D) it is accompanied with a sign of chronic diarrhea

HERE ARE THE SYMPTOMS OF PERSON HAVING IBS-D

- They will stool frequently
- It will look as if during your bowel movement, you are unable to empty it
- You will experience Sudden feeling/desire to have bowel movement

➢ You will experience pain in your abdomen

➢ You may also experience gas

❖ IBS accompanied with constipation(IBS-C) it is accompanied with a sign of abdominal pain

HERE ARE THE SYMPTOMS OF PERSON HAVING IBS-C

➢ They will stool frequently

- It will look as if during your bowel movement, you are unable to empty it
- When bowel movement is about to occur, it is straining
- You will experience Sudden feeling/desire to have bowel movement but are not possible
- You will experience pain in your abdomen

➢ You may also experience gas

➢ You may also experience bloating

To diagonise IBS, it must be up to six month duration. This diagnosis is done only when the rate at which you experience this signs are a minimum of three times a month.
There is an approved blood test that can help identify the existence of IBS in my body.

There is no special cure or food to remove IBS. many treatment that are available are only to reduce the symptoms. Everybody has their own body adaptation to food intake so we must know what food we eat that brings up IBS symptoms in the body. since everybody responds different to food, it is advisable to see your gastroenterologist for proper guide on what to eat so as to manage the ailment.

CHAPTER TWO

IRRITABLE BOWEL SYNDROME VERSUS INFLAMMATORY BOWEL SYNDROME.

Irritable bowel syndrome versus inflammatory bowel syndrome may have symptoms that are alike which are:

- They will stool frequently

- It will look as if during your bowel movement,

you are unable to empty

it

You will experience pain in

your abdomen

> You may also experience

gas

The irritable bowel syndrome is
highly different from
inflammatory bowel syndrome

In these aspect.

IBD is a combination of several
diseases among which are

Ulcerative and Crohns. These IBD is more severe than IBS.

IBS is not a disease but a gastrointestinal disorder and it comprises of combinations of different symptoms this is the reason why it is termed Syndrome and always taken as not too serious as compared to IBD.

Some symptoms that occur in IBD that are not found in IBS are:

- ✓ Rectal Bleeding
- ✓ Inflammatory Bowel disease
- ✓ Ulcers

Some things that can cause IBS since the main causes are unknown are:

- Increase Sensitivity to pain.
- Abnormal nervous system.
- Poor absorption of food.

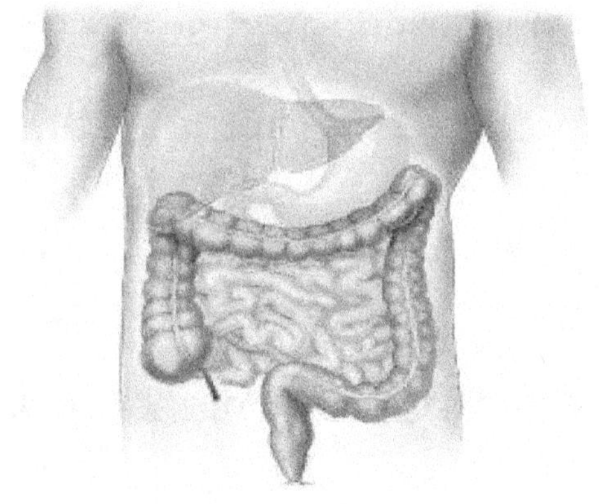

CHAPTER THREE

THE APPROVED TEST FOR IRRITABLE BOWEL SYNDROME (IBS)

When the test of IBS is to be carried out, other gastrointestinal disorder which may have symptoms that are similar are excluded. The doctor will do a total physical and verbal examination so as to be able to know how long such symptoms are in the persons body before carrying out any test.

The blood test Doctor will allow are test for :

1. CT SCAN
2. STOOL
3. X-RAY

These tests will be carried out and can be used to diagnose other problem and not any problem related to IBS.

There is a new discovered blood test that has shown that irritable bowel syndrome can be diagnosed. Example of such test is the irritable bowel syndrome with diarrhea(IBS-D) and the other one is the irritable bowel syndrome with combination of diarrhea and constipation(IBS-M) or It is sometimes called irritable bowel syndrome mixed

All of these tests can only diagnose the antibodies that are caused by several bacteria.

The rapid growth of these bacteria will speed up a heavy attack on the intestinal tissues of the person having that ailment. With such attack on the tissues of the intestine, the symptoms of IBS will be shown.

It is very important that antibody test be carried out because it helps to diagnose IBS-D and not IBS-C. The test becomes appropriate when the antibodies are fully discovered (present) therefore it will be traceable that IBS may be present. There are cases were the patient antibody might not be visible by test but yet the person has IBS ,such persons has to go for a higher and better testing which might be very expensive . the medical practitioner might refer the patient to a digestive system specialist to be diagnosed of upper endoscopy or may also be colonoscopy tested.

NOTE: Most women are subjected to having several

symptoms of IBS on or during their menstrual cycle.

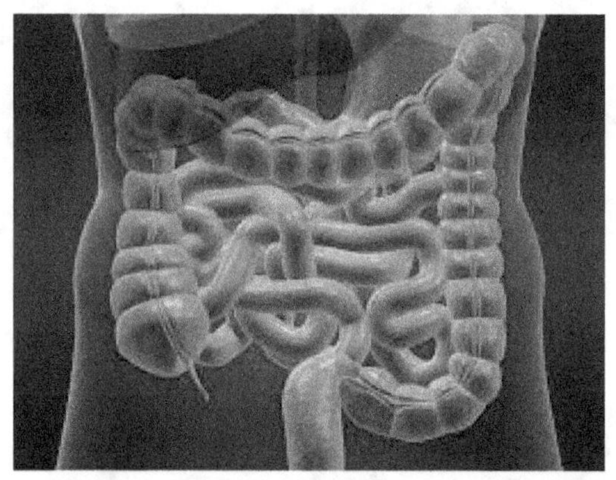

CHAPTER FOUR

IRRITABLE BOWEL SYNDROME, MEDICATIONS THAT TREAT (IBS-C) CONSTIPATION AND (IBS-D) DIARRHEA.

<u>DIARRHEA</u>

- ❖ It is recommended that female experiencing diarrhea should take Alosetron .You should take Rifaximin if you are experiencing bloating.

* ❖ Those experiencing loose of stool as their main difficulty should take: Loperamide and diphenoxylate

CONSTIPATION

Constipations are treated with these special drugs which are: Lubriprostone and Linaclotide

Bowel movement can be relieve with bisacodyl

(Dulcolax) and psyllium seed husks .

These drugs may trigger IBS attack with persons having (IBS-D) and good for patients with (IBS-C), Fluoxetine(Prozac),Citalopram(Celexa) and paroxetine(Paxil).

MOST PAIN AND CRAMPING EXPERIENCE IN IRRITABLE BOWEL SYNDROME (IBS) CAN BE TREATED WITH:

❖ ANTISPASMODICS: This help in the decreasing of

pain and cramping symptoms? such drugs are: Metoclopramide(Reglan),Dic yclomine(Bentyl)

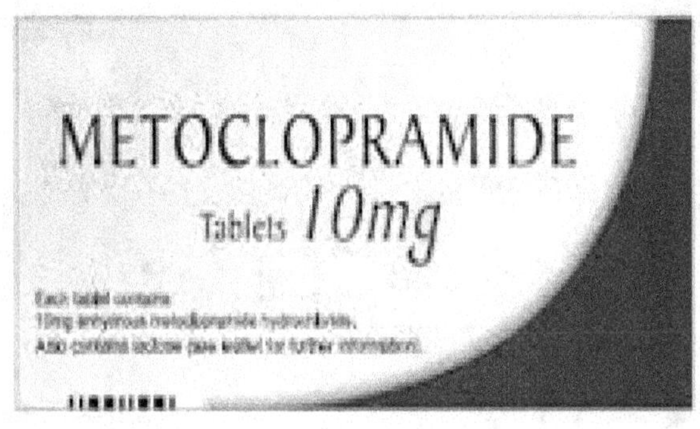

❖ Another is known as Antidepressants which are: Amitriptyline(Elavil,paregoric),nortriptyline(pamelor),and desipramine(Norpramin).

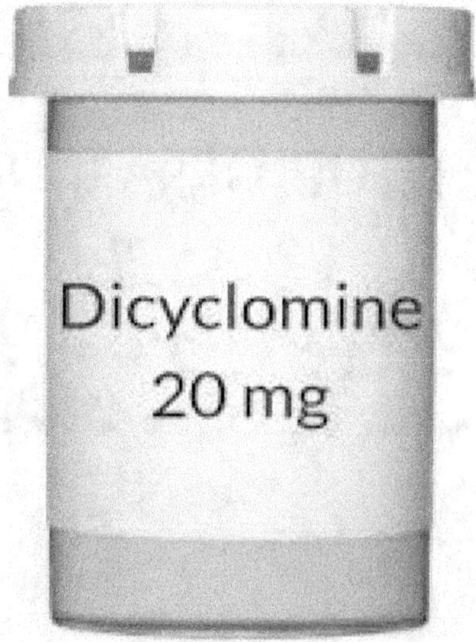

CHAPTER FIVE

THE APPROVED FOOD/HOME REMEDIES THAT IS GOOD FOR IBS PATIENTS.

The approved food that may provide relief for SOME PEOPLE ARE;

1. Good water intake
2. Taking food low of fat

3. Taking food high of carbonhydrate among which are pasta,whole grain bread and brown rice.

Most people has said that Kefil or Aloe Vera Juice are very good in reducing the symptoms.But in all it is advicable to see and tell your doctor before taking any one of these.

In some person, high intake of fiber food will help to reduce the symptoms of constipation in IBS cases,it may also cause another   worsen   harm   of bloating and gas.

Daily dosage intake of fiber food is 20grams to 35grams. Intake of fibre food lesser than this directed gram will have only to benefit from small increase in fibre. The amount of fibre in your diet should be increase gradually so as to reduce gas.

FOOD YOU MUST AVOID AS A PATIENT OF IBS ARE:

i. Fried or Fatty food

ii.   Dairy food (product): such diary product includes cheese and milk.

iii. Some vegetable that can cause increase in gas among which are broccoli, cabbage and legume beans.

iv.   Caffeine and Alcohol

v.   Food that are very high in sugar content

vi.   Chewing gums.

The Foundation for Functional Gastrointestinal Disorders,Inc. has been able to advice patients on food to eat and food not to eat.there you must see your doctor before you take any food as an IBS patients.

HOME AND NATURAL REMEDIES COMBINE WITH SOME LIFE STYLE PATTERN THAT MAY ASSIST IBS SYMPTOMS.

a) Eat smaller food and make it frequent

b) You must quit smoking

c) You must take regular exercise such as walking

d) Make sure you practice stress management and relaxation pattern

e) You should try and take ginger and

peppermint which help
to speed up digestion.

f) Learn and practice to
observe adequate
sleep.

g) Make sure you do not
take Laxative unless it
is directed to be taking
by your doctor.

ONLINE SITE TO GET IBS

www.medicinenet.com

www.webmd.com

www.nhs.uk

www.medlineplus.gov